Foods And Supplements For Arthritis

Pain Relief The Natural Way

Robert Lewis

Foods And Supplements For Arthritis

DEDICATION

To Tracey, my wife and best friend whose love and support is constant.

<u>Disclaimer</u>

The dietary suggestions in this book have been used by the author without ill effect.
However if the reader is taking medication it is wise to check with a doctor or health professional for any possible contraindications before taking supplements.

Suggestions for adding foods to your diet, should be safe unless you have a known allergy to them.

The recommendations in the book are for education and information only and not as medical advice.

Always keep supplements safe from children and infants.

The author and publisher accepts no liability.

CONTENTS

ACKNOWLEDGMENTS

Cover Picture: Alleksana, Courtesy, Pexels.com

<u>Introduction</u>

This short book was written to help fellow Arthritis sufferers and is based purely on my own experience and research into trying to alleviate my own pain from Osteoarthritis.

It is in no way to be considered a professional research document and any advice given herein is based purely on my own experiences. If you are unsure about any of the content, then please consult with your medical professional.

Most of the advice here relates to Osteoarthritis rather than Rheumatoid Arthritis but during research I have found that many of the suggestions may well help RA suffers also.

However I have found great relief by following the suggestions for diet and supplementation in this book.

I sincerely hope this helps you too.

Robert Lewis.

<u>Chapter 1</u>

My Own Pain Relief Journey

I don't remember when I started to notice pain or discomfort in my left knee and neck.
However I distinctly remember I was living in France and my wife was working for short periods in England. I went to collect her at a Ferry Port and the first thing she said to me was why are you limping? I hadn't even noticed! I also remember coming gingerly down stairs in the morning thinking this must be part of getting old. C'est la vie!

At this time I decided to seek medical help and went to my Doctor in France. He sent me for X-Rays and yes the answer was arthritis in my knee and neck. Returning to my doctor he gave me some strong NSAIDS (Non-Steroidal Anti-inflammatory Drug). I took these for a while and had some relief. I don't know why I didn't think to do it before but decided to research them a little on the internet.

The information I found worried me somewhat. Firstly the drug wasn't licensed in the UK. Secondly, I didn't like the sound of the potential side effects. Particularly liver damage.

Upon reflection I decided to try and find any natural/alternative remedies and see if I could improve my condition as I really didn't want to take drugs for my arthritis for ever more. My doctor also told me that if my condition worsened I may need an operation.

Rewind in time. My Mother introduced me to the benefits of
MSM (dietary sulphur).
I had Back pain from playing sport. So I decided to start
taking it again as it helped me then. My next breakthrough
was the addition of Rose Hips to my diet. This is one thing
that has reduced my discomfort enormously. These two
things plus adding Pineapple, Apples and Kiwi Fruit to my
regime have enabled me to live life without great discomfort.

 I tend to Power Walk mostly these days for exercise with
some intermittent sprints. I still get some discomfort but a
fraction of what it used to be. I think most Osteoarthritis
sufferers notice a change in the weather. Colder, damper for
instance can bring on the old aches but it only lasts for a few
days normally.

Chapter 2

The Reason For Pain

There can be several reasons for arthritis pain but here we can only deal with the main cause. Inflammation. Sounds obvious doesn't it. Logically, reduce inflammation and you reduce pain.

A protein called Fibrin goes towards the site of inflammation. Fibrin is used for blood clotting in the body but can build up excessively in our arthritic joints. To regulate the amount of Fibrin we have Proteolytic enzymes in our body. The problem is that as we age the amount of these important enzymes decreases. Ever wondered why young people don't have joint problems or that they heal quickly?

Fortunately we can address this problem through our diet. More on this later but for now it's important to recognise that some foods are bad for our arthritis and some are especially good.

https://www.sciencedaily.com/releases/2007/11/071116094750.htm

Chapter 3

First The Bad News

The following are foods that if you are eating too much of are going to cause inflammation.

Sugar

Sadly if you have too much in your diet then this can cause you problems with your arthritis. Most of us consume a certain amount of sugar in one form or another.
It is hidden in many processed foods and often when foods are labelled low fat they have more sugar in them. The problem is that fat in foods gives flavour and to compensate manufacturers often add sugar to make them taste nice. Personally I have a sweet tooth and find it difficult to reduce my intake but I use a natural sweetener called Stevia (made from the Stevia leaf) in drinks. It can be sprinkled on anything where you need that sweet taste. Try to limit sugary sodas and canned drinks.

https://www.medicalnewstoday.com/articles/326386

Gluten

Gluten in Bread, Pasta, Bagels, Muffins, Cakes. It is well known to cause inflammation of the gut and will affect your joints also. My wife is gluten intolerant and didn't know it for many years. Fortunately now you can buy many gluten free alternatives in shops. And some of them actually taste fine. I now eat gluten free pasta, and Nachos even though it's not necessary for me.

https://www.arthritis-health.com/types/general/how-gluten-can-cause-joint-pain

https://www.arthritis.org/health-wellness/healthy-living/nutrition/anti-inflammatory/the-connection-between-gluten-and-arthritis

Alcohol

Sadly alcohol is inflammatory as well. Try to keep your consumption moderate.
If you have to drink every day, just make it the one and maybe two on the week-end.
Better still just the week-end.

https://www.arthritis.org/health-wellness/healthy-living/nutrition/foods-to-limit/alcohol

Chips/French Fries and Processed Foods

The oil that is used for fries can cause inflammation. Too many trans fats are no good.
Major on Omega 3's rather than Omega 6's

https://www.arthritis-health.com/blog/difference-between-omega-3-and-omega-6-and-knee-arthritis-pain

Barbecued or Blackened foods

Heat destroys Proteolytic Enzymes. Don't eat these too often.

http://blog.arthritis.org/living-with-arthritis/high-cooking-temperature-inflammation/

To sum up, foods in their raw state are better for you because they have all their natural enzymes to fight pain.

Chapter 4

Now For The Good News

The following is a list of foods and extracts that will help fight inflammation.
I don't pretend this is an exhaustive list and I wouldn't expect anyone to include them all in their diet. I certainly don't.

Later I will tell you the foods and supplements I take to alleviate my arthritis. The first Five I consider to be the most important but if you can incorporate any of these it should help. Just a note that if you are going to try adding something to your diet particularly supplements. Give it a chance to work. Certain supplements take time to get into your system properly (Rose hips for instance)

Pineapple (Bromelaine-a mixture of enzymes that reduce inflammation)
Papaya   (Papain)
Rose Hips (Rosa Canina)
Kiwi Fruit
Apples (Rutin-Bioflavinoid that helps collagen production and utilisation of vitamin C)
Cherries
Ginger
Onions
Boswellia Extract
Coconut Oil
Extra Virgin Olive Oil & Olives
Pomegranates
MSM (Dietary Sulphur)
Oranges, Lemons, Limes (Citric Bioflavonoids)
Turmeric
Live Yogurt
Asparagus

On coconut oil, there have been studies on animals suggesting it has anti-inflammatory effects but no human trials I am aware of. So a little in your diet may be beneficial.

Chapter 5

Glucosamine

It seems the jury is still out on Glucosamine. Some studies seem to find that it helps a little with osteoarthritis whilst others don't. Take a look at this page at healthline.com

https://www.healthline.com/nutrition/glucosamine-and-arthritis

There are various links on this page that will take you to these studies if you want to dig deeper. These studies on various athletes seem to indicate improvement of symptoms whilst taking the supplement but when stopped there was no improvement.

Personally I don't take it although some people take a combination of msm and Glucosamine. More on MSM (dietary sulphur) in Chapter 6.

Chapter 6

<u>MSM</u>

MSM stands for Methylsulfonylmethane.
It's found in many foods including fresh fruits, meats and vegetables.
It has been found to reduce joint pain and swelling. It has a role in forming Collagen and Glucosamine needed for healthy joints and is claimed to have anti-inflammatory properties.

It seems that taken 50/50 with Glucosamine has the most benefit for joint mobility

I take MSM three times a day with meals.

It also is great for your skin and hair. Maybe that's why I look so young (ha ha)
I have seen a video on youtube that claims it makes your hair grow thicker and faster.
Not sure if that's true though!

https://www.versusarthritis.org/about-arthritis/complementary-and-alternative-treatments/types-of-complementary-treatments/msm/?gclid=EAIaIQobChMIlvifucHH6AIVyLHtChogdAdMEAAYASAAEgJc7_D_BwE

Chapter 7

Rose Hips

Rose Hips contain lycopene an anti-oxidant and high levels of vitamin C.
The most interesting substance though is a compound in the pulp called GoPo (glycoside of mono and diglycerol). The Rose Hip story began with a Danish farmer called Erik Hansen in the 1980's. He was given some pickled rose hips or rose hip marmalade and was intrigued by the health benefits. Being a farmer he decided to develop his own method of processing rose hips so the active substances were not lost. At first the rose hips were collected in the wild but this was not enough so he decided to grow his own. The rest is history as Hyben Vital Aps is now a global company and the product is marketed in the UK as GoPo.

For non-uk residents a google search for Hyben Vital should find you a distributor in your country.

The concentrated Rose Hips that are GoPo are the best that I have found. Below are some links to information pages about them.

https://www.rosehip-gopo.co.uk/about-gopo.html

http://www.gopo.co.uk/joint-health/

https://www.rosehip-gopo.co.uk/gopo-evidence.html

As mentioned before, it's important to give it time to really get into your system.
Take the recommended dose for at least 3 weeks before deciding if it works for you.

They aim to reduce joint pain, improve mobility and reduce the need for painkillers.
I urge you to try them but get the best quality available to you. This will be dependent on where you live, shops, delivery etc.

Chapter 8

Cherries

Although not so readily available in supermarkets, cherries can be another great food weapon in our armoury.

Cherries contain a flavonoid (anthocyanin) that may be attributed to it's anti-inflammatory effect. As well as Vitamin C they contain potassium, copper, manganese and are high in polyphenols.

Research suggests that Tart cherries particularly the Montmorency variety are the best for fighting inflammation. If you can't obtain cherries easily you might be able to find cherry juice, the next best thing.

Incidentally, they are allegedly very good for gout sufferers.

Look out for them when they are in your local food store.

Chapter 9

Proteolytic Enzymes

These enzymes perform many useful functions in our bodies. Namely digestion of protein, blood clotting, immune function, wound healing and tissue repair.

Some are produced naturally in our body. Pepsin, Trypsin and chymotrypsin are used in digestive processes. The ones we can gain extra benefit from are found in foods.

See the list in Chapter 4

The importance of these for arthritis sufferers is that they have an anti-imflammatory effect on our bodies. In particular they can dissolve Fibrin deposits and debris in our joints. This inflammation is one reason for our pain.

Some of the benefits are:

1) Reduce swelling

2) Improve circulation

3) Increase supply of nutrients to injured or damaged joints

4) Breakdown debris to facilitate easier removal from areas of wear and tear.

The subject of Proteolytic Enzymes is quite complex and greater investigation/explanation is not the intention of this self-help book.

However, I understand that medical science is continuing to investigate the uses of these amazing enzymes as a safe alternative to NSAID's (Non-steroidal Anti-inflammatory Drugs).

I have included some links to further information in the last chapter for further reading. Again, if the links do not work for any reason, just copy and paste the text link into your preferred web browser.

Chapter 10

Supplements I take

Vitamin C

Vitamin C is water soluble therefore can be taken safely. It was once described to me as a sponge full of water. When it's full it just drips out, much like your body you will pass it out. So it's unlikely that any of us will take it in so called "toxic" amounts.

Vitamin D

Most of us know that going out in the Sun can increase our vitamin D levels but only if the skin is exposed. We are more aware of the dangers of skin cancer these days though and people working in offices don't get the opportunity to take advantage of the Sun. Vitamin D it vital for healthy bones and teeth. It plays a role in the regulation of calcium and phosphorus levels in the blood.

Zinc

Known for boosting the immune system, best taken with vitamin C to help absorption.
Particularly good for Men as it helps produce the sex hormones testosterone and prolactin.

Beef Liver capsules (from Argentinian Grass Fed Cattle).

Liver was a popular supplement for body builders in the 70's and 80's before nutritional science went into overdrive. It has all the B vitamins as well as Iron, Vitamin A. A great supplement that has many claimed health benefits including boosting immune system and maintaining good cholesterol levels.

Kelp

Rich in many minerals and antioxidants, Vitamins A, C,K & E, Iodine, Iron, Potassium, Calcium, Magnesium & Copper. It's important to buy Kelp that grows in clean waters as if growing in polluted areas it can absorb heavy metals. Therefore not recommended for Pregnant or breast feeding women, children or people with kidney problems.
Much is made about the iodine content and uses as a thyroid supplement. It's probably not necessary if you have enough salt in your diet. Go easy, just 1 tablet a day if you want to get the trace mineral benefit.

Whether you decide to supplement or not is an individuals choice. Personally I don't mind if people don't agree with it. I have been taking supplements for the last 30 years or so and I am still here in relatively good health. In fact I am frequently told that I look young for my age (67 at the time of writing). As always the choice is yours just be sensible about the amounts.

<u>Chapter 11</u>

<u>Summary</u>

I have covered many foods and additives that may help you in your quest to be pain free from arthritis. Realistically you can't use or add them all to your diet.

Equally you don't have to eliminate all the bad foods from your diet completely. Just try and work out which ones are the inflammation triggers for you. Keeping a food diary may help in this respect.

However, if you just try some of these suggestions they may help you as much as they have helped me.

The supplements will unfortunately take a hit on your purse/wallet. Fruits however can be incorporated into your diet at less of an expense. My own feeling is that you can't put a price on your health/comfort. After all we only live once and as somebody once said:
the body you have is the best body you are going to get.

Therefore if money is tight my suggestion is try good quality Rose Hips and buy some Pineapple and Kiwi Fruit. Make a fruit salad from these two and store in the fridge.
You can eat some daily with your preferred option. I like mine with some live yogurt and crunchy oats or dry cereal sprinkled on top. Eat apples often also.

I hope the information herein helps you to reduce your pain/discomfort.

This book was orginally created for Kindle and contains many links to websites. These obviously wont work for a printed version. However if you email me at the adress below with Arthritis Links in the subject line, I will send you a pdf file with all the clickable links.

If you have found this short book useful, you can leave a review and/or email me at:

hack125448@yahoo.com

Best wishes

Robert Lewis

Chapter 12-Various Resources

Fibrin

https://www.sciencedaily.com/releases/2007/11/071116094750.htm

https://www.jci.org/articles/view/30134

Proteolytic Enzymes

https://nutritionreview.org/2013/04/controlling-inflammation-proteolytic-enzymes

http://www.specialtyenzymes.com/blog/Proteolytic-Enzymes-Help-with-Inflammation

Rose Hips

https://www.ncbi.nlm.nih.gov/pmc/articles/PMC5485961

https://www.rosehip-gopo.co.uk/about-gopo.html

http://www.gopo.co.uk/joint-health

https://www.rosehip-gopo.co.uk/gopo-evidence.html

General

https://www.thehealthy.com/arthritis/foods-bad-for-arthritis

Pineapple (Bromelaine)

https://www.ncbi.nlm.nih.gov/pmc/articles/PMC538506

Papaya (Papain)

https://www.verywellhealth.com/the-benefits-of-papain-89493

Kiwi Fruit

https://www.medicalnewstoday.com/articles/271232

Ginger

https://www.ncbi.nlm.nih.gov/pmc/articles/PMC3665023

http://blog.arthritis.org/living-with-arthritis/health-benefits-of-ginger

Onions

http://blog.arthritis.org/living-with-arthritis/onions-prevent-inflammation-arthritis-diet

https://www.onions-usa.org/onionista/onions-inflammation-superfood

Boswellia Extract (Check possible side effects and with doctor if taking meds)

https://www.healthline.com/health/boswellia

https://www.ncbi.nlm.nih.gov/pmc/articles/PMC3309643

Extra Virgin Olive Oil & Olives

https://www.chatelaine.com/health/diet/five-health-benefits-of-olives-and-olive-oil-plus-a-zesty-tapenade-recipe

https://www.healthline.com/nutrition/13-anti-inflammatory-foods

Pomegranates (The fruit is ok but supplements may react with meds, so check with doctor)

https://www.healthline.com/health/rheumatoid-arthritis/rheumatoid-arthritis-pomegranate

https://www.ncbi.nlm.nih.gov/pmc/articles/PMC5622718

Cherries

https://www.arthritis.org/health-wellness/healthy-living/nutrition/healthy-eating/best-fruits-for-arthritis

http://blog.arthritis.org/living-with-arthritis/arthritis-diet-cherries

https://www.healthline.com/nutrition/cherries-benefits

https://health.usnews.com/health-news/blogs/eat-run/2015/03/23/10-foods-that-fight-inflammation

Sugar

https://www.medicalnewstoday.com/articles/326386

Gluten

https://www.arthritis-health.com/types/general/how-gluten-can-cause-joint-pain

Gluten

https://www.arthritis.org/health-wellness/healthy-living/nutrition/anti-inflammatory/the-connection-between-gluten-and-arthritis

Alcohol

https://www.arthritis.org/health-wellness/healthy-living/nutrition/foods-to-limit/alcohol

Processed Foods

https://www.arthritis-health.com/blog/difference-between-omega-3-and-omega-6-and-knee-arthritis-pain

Barbecued Foods

http://blog.arthritis.org/living-with-arthritis/high-cooking-temperature-inflammation/

Glucosamine

https://www.healthline.com/nutrition/glucosamine-and-arthritis

MSM

https://www.versusarthritis.org/about-arthritis/complementary-and-alternative-treatments/types-of-complementary-treatments/msm/?gclid=EAIaIQobChMIlvifucHH6AIVyLHtChogdAdMEAAYASAAEgJc7_D_BwE

 As always with the ever changing World Wide Web, web pages come and go. At the time of writing all the links were working.
Sites or even web pages are taken down from time to time. Apologies anyway if any of them are not working.

Robert Lewis

ABOUT THE AUTHOR

Robert Lewis lives in a seaside town on the South Coast of
England.
After living in France for 14 years and exploring in his Motor
home decided to return to his roots.
He enjoys building computers, long walks by the sea, his
wife's cooking and has promised to go sea fishing one day.
An interest in food supplements for better health helps to
keep him young!